The Anti-Inflammatory Diet & Action Plans

—

14-Day Meal Plan and Proven Recipes to Heal Your Inflammation Disease - Finally Alleviate Pain, Heal Your Immune System and Restore Your Overall Health

By Abigail Murphy

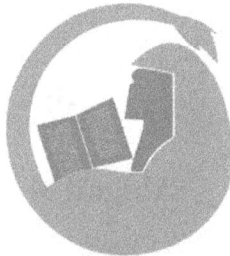

EFFINGO
Publishing

For more great books visit:

EffingoPublishing.com

The Anti-Inflammatory Diet & Action Plans—

02 Week Meal Plan and Proven Delicious Recipes to Heal Your Inflammation Disease - Finally, Alleviate Pain, Heal Your Immune System and Restore Your Overall Health

By:

Abigail Murphy

Download another book for Free

We want to thank you for purchasing this book and offer you another book (just as long and valuable as this book), "Health & Fitness Mistakes You Don't Know You're Making", completely free.

Visit the link below to signup and receive it:

www.effingopublishing.com/gift

In this book, we will break down the most common health & fitness mistakes, you are probably committing right now, and will reveal how you can easily get in the best shape of your life!

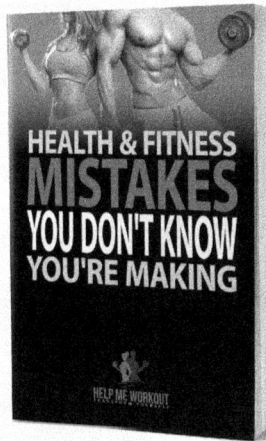

In addition to this valuable gift, you will also have an opportunity to get our new books for free, enter giveaways, and receive other valuable emails from us. Again, visit the link to sign up:

www.effingopublishing.com/gift

TABLE OF CONTENTS

Introduction

The internet is full of scientific shreds of evidence that proves that eating healthy food is packed with healing powers. Today, we have observed that chronic diseases become the most common elements in our life. Every other person is suffering from conditions like heart diseases, Blood-Pressure, Arthritis, Diabetes & many others.

All such diseases have a strong relevance with "Chronic Inflammation." It's a type of disease in which the organs of the body are inflamed, along with causing inflammation in blood vessels, brain, and joints in the body.

The purpose of writing this book is to help people suffering from such disease by providing adequate action plans. The book intends to provide all the relevant information to people who may think or have inflammation disease. With the help of this book, they will be able to identify if they are suffering from such a chronic illness.

The book contains a series of actions for people suffering from Chronic Disease for them to follow to help their situation. The book includes a 14-day Meal Plan & delicious recipes to heal inflammation disease.

Also, before you get started, I recommend you joining our email newsletter to receive updates on any upcoming new book releases or promotions. You can sign-up for free, and as a bonus, you will receive a free gift. Our "*Health & Fitness Mistakes You Don't Know You're Making*" book! This book has been written to demystify, expose the top do's and don'ts and to finally equip you with the information you need to get in the best shape of your life. Due to the overwhelming amount of mis-information and lies told by magazines and self-proclaimed "gurus", it's becoming harder and harder to get reliable information to get in shape. Instead of going through dozens of biased, unreliable and un-trustworthy sources to get your health & fitness information, we have broken down all the information that you need in this book for you to easily follow and immediately get results to achieve your desired fitness goals in the shortest amount of time.

Once again, to join our email newsletter and to receive a free copy of this valuable book, please visit the link and signup now: www.effingopublishing.com/gift

Chapter 01: What is

Inflammation & Auto-Immunity

The inflammation in the body is the process in which the body fights against cells that are harmful to it. It's a body's natural way to heal itself after fighting with certain infections, wounds, and other toxic chemicals present in the body.

So, inflammation is healthy for a body as it repairs the damaged cells. If the inflammatory actions occur in the body when it is not needed, it becomes an unsettled situation that leads to many other diseases in the body.

If left untreated, this chronic disease affects Heart, Blood-Vessels, Brain tissues & many other organs of the body. There are many ways of treating the body's unwanted inflammation. One of the easiest & healthiest ways of treating inflammation is to adapt to the Anti-Inflammatory Diet. Food is believed to provide the body with all the necessary elements that are required by the body to heal itself. By adopting a healthy diet & a healthy lifestyle, we can keep the inflammation at the surface.

Have you ever thought of the causes of inflammation in the body? There are many reasons for inflammation to occur in a body. The reasons include unhealthy nutrition, toxins in the environment, genetics, lack of any physical activity, dependency on any medication, anxiety, and stress.

To have a better understanding, let me draw a comparison between Inflammation & Fire. If used in a limited or controlled portion, fire is essential to keep us warm, healthy, and covered. If it is not controlled or used in limited portions, it can have lethal effects on the body. Also, it doesn't have to be big to cause destruction. Thus, inflammation is also healthy for the body; it's a natural repair system of the body. If it occurs in a place where it is not needed, then it starts affecting the overall body.

Although, by having a healthy diet, you can take charge of your health. As mentioned, Inflammation in the body is a protective action of the body against the infections. However, by adopting a healthy diet plan, we can convert this protective approach into preventive measures of the body to stay away from such a chronic disease.

Auto-Immunity

The Auto-Immune system of a body is defined as the mechanism that intends to protect the body when exposed to bacteria, infections & tumor cells. However, the purpose is to save the body from different viruses. Still, if left uncontrolled, the immune system starts affecting the body's tissues & organs that become the prime factor of auto-immune diseases in the body.

Auto-Immune Diseases

Auto-Immune Diseases includes a wide span of diseases that have the power to affect different organs of the body. The inflammation is strongly correlated with auto-immune diseases. The Auto-Immune Diseases are classified based on affected parts of the body. Type 01 is known as Localized Autoimmune Diseases; such conditions are confined to specific organs and tissues.

Some of the examples of Confined Autoimmune Diseases are

- *Addison's Disease*

This disease damages the outer part of the adrenal gland making the autoimmunity as the prime cause. In this disease, a person's adrenal glands do not make sufficient hormones that result in weakness, dullness, and inappropriate diet. If left untreated, the disease can become lethal.

- *Grave's Disease*

It's a disease that affects a person's thyroid. This disease is known as the most important factor to cause "Hyperthyroidism," resulting in excessive production of antibodies that generate a false warning for the Thyroid Gland to produce needless hormones.

- *Type-1 Diabetes*

Type-1 is a medical condition in which a person's pancreas doesn't produce enough insulin for the normal working of the organ. If left untreated, this disease leads to severe health problems as insulin is essentially required to control the levels of blood sugar.

- *Crohn's Disease*

It's a type of inflammatory disease that affects a person's digestive system. Some of the symptoms are dullness, pain in the abdomen, and weakness in the body.

Types of Inflammation

Acute Inflammation

The inflammation takes place in the body as a result of a bruise on the leg, a twisted ankle, or a sore throat is called Acute Inflammation. It is a short-term defense mechanism, in which inflammation in the body occurs in the body at a place where it is needed. The significant effects of Acute Inflammation are redness, pain in the affected place, and also the organ stops working only under severe cases.

In acute inflammation, the blood vessels expand, with the increased blood flow, and the white blood cells in the body move towards the damaged area to support fast recovery. As a result, the damaged area becomes swollen and red.

Acute Inflammation is responsible for releasing the chemical named "Cytokines." The chemical is released by the affected tissue of the organ and works as an "Alarming Signal." These warning signals allows your auto-immune system to heal the damaged organ.

Also, certain substances like prostaglandins are responsible for blood clotting to heal the affected organ. That's why pain & fever becomes part of the healing process. When the body starts healing, the symptoms of Acute Inflammation tends to descend.

Chronic Inflammation

This inflammation takes place in a body when it is not needed. It's a long-term defense mechanism and constant inflammation. Chronic Inflammation leads to many other diseases. Such type of inflammation is a threat to a body as it occurs in a place where it is not needed.

The White-Blood Cells that are responsible for defending the body against any viruses or infections tend to gather at a place internally. When they don't see any damage, they had nowhere to go; hence they start damaging the body internally.

Also, they become responsible for developing other diseases in the body. That's why we need to adopt a healthy lifestyle to stay away from such a chronic disease.

From children to adults, everybody is prone to Inflammation in the body

Certain health conditions that are linked with the inflammation include

➢ *Heart Disease*

Inflammation is the biggest threat to the Cardiovascular System. As per the research, heart problems become the most significant cause of deaths for the people living in the United States of America. The higher levels of inflammation in the body lead to a heart attack or stroke.

Chronic Inflammation leads to the expansion of your blood vessels. The expansion of blood vessels leads to blood-clotting, which becomes the leading cause of a heart attack or stroke.

If blood-clotting occurs in an artery of heart, a person suffers heart-attack. Likewise, if blood-clotting occurs in any of the brain arteries, a person suffers a stroke.

➢ *Inflammatory Bowel Disease (IBD)*

Inflammatory Bowel Disease occurs as a result of inflammation in the body. It's a disease that affects a person's digestive system. The type of disease is further classified into two types.

1) Ulcerative Colitis

It's a type of IBD that is responsible for higher levels of inflammation in the inner side of a person's large intestine

2) Crohn's IBD

It's a type of IBD that is responsible for an increased level of inflammation that affects the person's digestive system.

> *Obesity*

Obesity is another health condition that occurs as a result of inflammation in the body. As per the research, the disease rates have reached such a greater extent and around 2 billion people in the world are obese.

> *Rheumatoid Arthritis*

It's a chronic disease that causes extreme pain, inflexibility, and inflammation in the joints. The disease occurs when the immune system attacks the joints. It can also affect the heart & lungs. As per the research, more than 50 million people are suffering from this disease all over America.

> *Allergies*

Different allergies from food, medicines, and toxins present in the environment also become the main cause of Inflammation in the body. Many people are suffering from different allergies all over America.

➤ Asthma

When inflammation affects the lungs, it results in asthma & many other diseases related to the lungs. Some of the health conditions like cough, cold, improper breaths all are related to having inflammation on the lungs.

➤ Lupus

It's a medical condition that affects different parts of the body. Some of the prominent parts are Joints, Skin, heart-related health conditions, and lungs.

➤ Cancer

Inflammation can also become the main cause of cancer. The inflammation leads to abnormal growth of cells, and it is one of the main causes of deficiency of healthy cells from the body.

➤ Celiac Disease

It's a disease in which the body does not produce sufficient gluten, which results in damaging the small intestine.

➤ *Skin-Diseases*

The most common diseases that we took for granted are Skin-Diseases. Skin diseases occur as a result of inflammation in the organs inside the body. It includes Acne, eczema, tiny bumps, red patches, and psoriasis. If left untreated, these skin condition becomes the permanent part of an individual's skin and also lead to other skin related problems.

➤ *Headaches*

Another most common medical condition triggered as a result of inflammation is Headache. As per the research, more than 35 million people are suffering from a migraine all over America.

➤ *Neurological Disorders*

As per the research, it has been observed that neurological orders share a strong correlation with inflammation in different organs of the body.

Signs of Inflammation

Some of the symptoms of Inflammation are discussed in this section. The below mentioned are the scientifically proven symptoms of inflammation in the body.

1) Weariness

Either sleeping too much or having a little sleep can both lead to inflammation in the body. The average sleep recommended by the experts is between 6 to 8 hours. If you are following this routine of sleep and still feel weariness, then your body is probably suffering from inflammation. Being Fatigued Out has been observed as the most common symptom of inflammation. Despite having proper sleep, if you observe weariness, then you should consult the doctor

2) Severe Headaches.

The headaches are the most common indication of inflammation in the body. If you feel a continuous pain at the shoulders or the spine, chances are you are suffering from inflammation in the body.

3) Digestive difficulties

Most of the time, unwanted inflammation occurs around the stomach. It directly affects a person's digestive system. When the digestive system is affected, a person finds it hard to digest anything.

Besides, inflammation around the Stomach results in bloating, cramping, and other food allergies.

If you have observed a problem with your digestion, you should probably consult a doctor.

4) Swollen Lymph Nodes

The Lymph Nodes are present around your neck. These nodes serve a "HUB" to a person's immune system. You might have observed some swollen nodes in case of a cold or sore throat. You don't need to worry about recognizing such an issue; it means that your body is fighting against the virus. However, if the condition doesn't fade away on its own, then you should consult a doctor.

5) Stuffed Nose

It might sound weird, but Yes, Stuffed Nose is another indication of you having inflammation in the body. A body has different ways of reacting to inflammation. The issues like cold, watery eyes, and stuffed nose, are all related to having inflammation in the body.

6) Acne

The acne is the most common symptom of a body having internal inflammation. It's a medical condition that affects people of all ages. However, it goes away after some time, and there is no need to take medicines for acne. If you observe your acne stays for a more extended period, then you should consult a doctor to check if you are suffering from any other chronic disease.

7) Brain-Fog

The inflammation in the body can also affect the brain. Most of the people find it hard to think. We shouldn't take this for granted and consult a doctor because the inability to think is also another common sign of inflammation in the body.

8) Heartburn

Another latent indication of inflammation is heartburn in the body. It is quite hard to identify as many people confuse it with digestive issues. It's a medical condition in which the stomach acid travels up to the esophagus and causing severe heartburns.

Myths about Autoimmune Diseases

Many people have different opinions when it comes to having autoimmune diseases. Many people have strong beliefs that these autoimmune diseases cannot be cured even by adopting a different lifestyle.

So, we will discuss some of the myths about autoimmune diseases and analyze if there is any authenticity to these myths.

Disorders exist for the life-time

It's entirely true that if left untreated, these diseases can have adverse effects on a person's health for the whole lifetime. But, with the help of an anti-inflammatory diet, these disorders can be reversed.

Disorders can vanish only with the help strong medications

Autoimmune diseases occur as a result of inflammation in the body. However, in severe cases, a person has to undergo a thorough medical treatment. But, it has been significantly observed that by adopting an anti-inflammatory diet, the need to take strong medicines has reduced up to a greater extent.

Bad digestion has no relevance with inflammation

The myth of having no relevance to the digestive system with inflammation in the body is useless. Many types of research have been conducted in the past that shows a strong correlation of bad digestive system with inflammation.

You can't change your genetics

Yeah, we can't change our genetics, but we can control it. It has been observed that people having autoimmune disorders have shown significant improvement by adopting an anti-inflammatory diet. The genetics may count 30% of the chances, but 70% is based on the environment you surround yourself with. So, despite having these disorders in your genes, you can still manage to control these symptoms and have a better life.

Ways to Reduce Inflammation

Despite being the most severe medical condition, if left untreated, you will be surprised to know that inflammation can easily be controlled just by adopting a different lifestyle. The changed lifestyle not only helps you to control the inflammation in the body but also enables you to reduce the cholesterol and sugar levels of the body.

In this book, we will discuss in detail about having a positive lifestyle. However, some of the changes to reduce inflammation are mentioned below:

1) No Smoking.

Smoking is widely recognized to have been associated with the heart-diseases. It is the most common cause of damaging the lungs. The side effects of smoking are not only limited to heart and lung problems, but it also is one of the causes of inflammation in the body. It damages the person's blood vessels and also endorses atherosclerosis. So by quitting this habit, the chances of heart diseases are reduced to half.

2) Body Weight

As discussed above, obesity is another essential cause of inflammation in the body. The inability to maintain a body weight can decrease the risk factor for various diseases. Carrying a large amount of fat around your stomach is a warning for heart diseases. By maintaining a healthy body-weight, inflammation levels in the body are reduced up to significant extents.

3) Exercise

Lack of physical activity can lead not only to inflammation but also many other diseases. Exercising anywhere between 20 minutes to 60 minutes has the power to reduce inflammation in the body. Long-walks and sprint walks are also very effective in reducing the inflammation from the body.

4) Anti-Inflammatory Diet

The choice of food has a lot to do with reducing the inflammation in the body. Many people eat food that contains a large number of sugars and is processed. Eating such foods has adverse effects on health as they are primarily responsible for inflammation in the body. The Anti-inflammatory Diet, by far, proves to be the most effective yet the safest way of reducing inflammation.

Just by adding different fruits & vegetables to your diet, you can drastically reduce the higher levels of inflammation from the body.

5) Don't stress

The way you manage chronic stress has a lot to do with reducing the inflammation levels. With the help of different exercises, you can very well manage your stress

6) Avoid Sugars

Refined Sugar is considered as the most common cause of inflammation in the body. Despite it being associated with health risks, people have it throughout the day. You can have controlled inflammation just by avoiding or limiting the amount of sugar you take.

7) Proper Sleep

Sleeping is considered as the best repair therapy of a human body. It allows every part of your body to rest and repair itself. Undoubtedly, having a good sleep is linked to many health benefits. By having a proper sleep of between 6 to 8 hours, the levels of inflammation are greatly reduced.

Chapter 02: Heal Your Immune System & Your Overall Health

There are certain things in life that we have no control over. Luckily, we always have the option of controlling our diet. It's ultimately our personal choice to provide healthy nutrition to our body. Healthy nutrition plays a significant role in preventing, developing, managing, and controlling these inflammatory diseases.

One should be familiar enough with the types of food that are harmful to the body. There is a wide variety of food available on the market, and it's very convenient to pick healthy food. It doesn't matter if you are a vegan, or you are following a different diet plan, the important thing is to pick something healthy for the body and avoid these inflammatory diet plans.

So, the second chapter is dedicated to eating healthy food and healing your immune system and your overall health.

Foods that Aggravate Inflammation

The best medicine to heal your Immune system and your overall health is healthy food. The choices we make with foods can either heal inflammation or cause it to aggravate. In this section, we will discuss all such foods that have adverse effects on health, and we will also discuss ways to heal inflammation in the body.

1) Dairy Products

Dairy is generally considered as an essential food that is responsible for strengthening bones, and it helps in keeping us strong. Perhaps, it is good and healthy for many people, but to some, dairy is not a good food to eat. The human body is so complex, and it is made up of millions of enzymes, each with a different function. If anyone of these enzymes is not working properly, then it leads to various problems in the body.

Lactase is an enzyme that is present in the small intestine of human beings. The Lactase enzyme is very critical, and it is responsible for digesting dairy products that we consume.

However, there are some people with Lactase deficiency. Their bodies don't produce Lactase that is needed to digest "Lactose Sugars" in milk. The deficiency is not something we can take for granted. If left uncontrolled, it can also lead to gas, stomach problems, and diarrhea.

Besides Lactose Intolerance, there are many other allergies and diseases that a person can suffer by consuming Dairy Products.

As per the research conducted by FARE (Food, Allergy, Research, and Education), these chronic inflammatory diseases are very common in people living in North America.

Today, some people still believe that milk is mucus-forming food. The reason it obstructs digestion is that it creates a slime on the digestive path and stops healthy nutrition from being consumed or absorbed.

Dairy products are prepared from milk. The Cows to give milk for dairy products are raised with artificial growth hormones and medicines. When we consume such products, there are higher chances that these medicines and synthetic growth hormones can intervene with our hormones and can also lead to inflammatory diseases.

Also, Dairy products are loaded with tons of sugars, and artificial flavor for extra sweetness can also aggravate inflammation in the body.

The dairy products that you should not consume are

- Milk

- Yogurt

- Cheese

- Butter

- Ice-cream

- Kefir etc.

   2)   Gluten Products

The next is Gluten, which is found to have many adverse health effects on the body. It is found in wheat, barley, triticale, and some other products. Gluten helps foods like cereal, pasta, and bread in holding their shapes.

Also, Gluten is also found in some of the cosmetic products like lip balm and glue on the back of envelopes.

Gluten Intolerance has also become one of the common health problems for people living in the United States. The people suffering from such a disease find it hard to digest gluten at all. A diet plan that includes Gluten and its products can lead to severe health problems for people suffering from it.

As per the research, it has been observed that around 35 % of adults in the U.S have decided to cut gluten from their diet. Also, some of them don't have Celiac disease. Still, to be on the safer side, people have decided to cut gluten from their diet.

Besides, it has also been observed that processed food contains "hidden gluten." The people who want to have a gluten-free diet should check the labels mentioning, "Gluten-Free" before buying these processed foods.

Let's take an example of Oats. During the formation of oats, they come into contact with Wheat, and it's not at all healthy for a person who has Celiac disease.

People with Celiac disease can be so sensitive, that even small traces of gluten in any of their foods can make their condition worse. So, they have to be very careful while eating something. Besides, some of the non-edible items can also contain gluten in it, and people with Celiac disease should stay away from such products. Some of the non-edible foods with gluten are :

- Lipsticks, and lip balms for chapped lips
- Food supplements

As mentioned earlier, Gluten is used in the products to hold their shapes. It is a hidden ingredient; that's why people with Celiac disease should be very cautious while buying gluten-free foods. Some of the foods with Gluten that we all should avoid are:

- Cake
- Candies
- Pieces of bread
- Noodles

- Soups

- Bakery items

- Soy

  3) Peanuts

The health effects of these foods vary from person to person. Some people are not allergic to peanuts, but some people are prone to different allergies while consuming Peanuts. However, peanuts contain omega-6 fatty acids, and much other healthy nutrition, still, one must avoid eating peanuts to stay safe from these chronic inflammatory diseases. Also, peanut butter and other peanut products in the market use artificial flavors and lots of sugar, which can create many health-related problems in the body.

2) Alcohol Consumption

If consumed in limits, it may provide an individual with different antioxidants. But, if consumed excessively, it can lead to producing "C-reactive Protein."

One of the common problems that people who consume alcohol can face is "Leaky Gut." It's a disease in which the body encounters problems with different bacterial toxins roaming out of the colon and in the body. Hence, Leaky-Gut is responsible for having inflammation in the body.

3) Corns

Corn is the most common GMO food. Almost 85 % of the corn in the United States is "Genetically Modified, or engineered food." GMO foods are the foods that are specifically produced by the organisms, with changes in the DNAs using genetic engineering methods. So these GMO foods are comparatively new for our metabolism and can impose serious health effects. These modifications are not suitable for health. Corn products such as vegetable oil, corn sugar, corn syrup are all very rich in Omega-6 fatty acids and are the main cause of inflammation in the body.

Some of the corn foods to avoid are:

- Maltose
- Corn Syrup
- Golden Syrup
- Corn Starch
- Corn Sugar

- Corn flour

6) Soy

Like Corn, soy is also considered as one of the most common allergens. It also falls under the category of GMO foods. As per the research, around 90 percent of the soy used in the United States of America is genetically engineered. Also, the food contains goitrogens that are primarily responsible for obstructing thyroid function. The anti-nutrients that are present in it can also interact with the digestive system and causes inflammation. Some of the soy foods to avoid are:

- Tofu

- Soy yogurt

- Soy protein

- Soy ice-cream

- Flour

- Oils

7) Caffeine

Caffeine has been recognized as the morning booster and is consumed by people all over the world. It's a chemical compound that is found tea and coffee. But if you are suffering from the inflammatory disease, then caffeine is a bad option for you. The chemical compound interacts with the digestion system and obstructs your digestion process resulting in inflammation. Along with just digestive problems, caffeine is also known for increasing heartbeats, eating disorders, and it can also increase a person's blood pressure. Although it is used all over the world, it doesn't justify the side-effects of this chemical compound.

4) Sugar

Undoubtedly, sugar is harmful to health. It is also referred to as "White Poison" it increases blood-sugar levels, which leads to the production of Inflammatory-Cytokines. Artificial flavors, sweeteners, and processed foods contain tons of sugar in it. It damages bones and weakens the immune system.

5) Eggs

It might sound strange, but Yes, Eggs are also inflammatory to some people, and they find it hard to digest it. It has been observed that feedlot eggs are rich in Omega 6-fatty acids, which is responsible for inflammation in the body. On the other hand, organic eggs are loaded with healthy nutrition and Omega 3 fatty acids that are incredibly healthy for our bodies.

6) Nightshade Vegetables

Nightshade Vegetables belong to a particular plant family named "Solanaceae" Some of these species are toxic, such as the belladonna plant, which is considered as the poisonous nightshade. However, human beings also eats others ones including white potatoes, tomatoes, paprika, eggplant, bell-pepper.

The reason these vegetables are considered harmful because they have alkaloid in them, and that is very toxic for the body. It is also believed that these vegetables are strongly correlated with causing inflammation in the body.

Foods to eat to have a healthy body

In the above section, we have discussed the foods that aggravate inflammation in the body. It might appear to you that there is nothing left to eat, and every other food is related to inflammation. That's certainly not the case, even after avoiding the foods mentioned above, there is still plenty of foods to eat to have a healthy body.

The vegetables and fruits are known as the best anti-inflammatory foods. These are the food loaded with healthy nutrition and can drastically reduce inflammation from the body.

1) Apple-Cider Vinegar

Many people underestimate the qualities of Apple-Cider Vinegar. It is made up of apples after the fermentation process. It dramatically increases the acid levels in the stomach and improves digestion. As we have seen that most of these inflammatory diseases occur as a result of poor digestion. When we use Apple-Cider Vinegar, it not only helps in digestion but also saves us from cold, coughs, flu, and other bacterial infections.

2) Bone Broths

Bone Broths are liquids containing bones and connective tissues. It is very beneficial for the inflammation and very easy to make. It contains collagen and other healthy nutrition, a vitamin for the body. Also, it offers plenty of amino acids for the body. The amino acids present in it are known to help the digestion process. As per the research, people having a problem with digestion tend to have reduced levels of Amino acids in the body. The bone broths are one of the safest and healthiest ways of increasing the amino acid levels in the body.

3) Fish

Red meat has a bad reputation when it comes to a healthy body. The reason for its bad reputation is cholesterol; that is one of the reasons for aggravating inflammation. Whereas Fish meat has earned an excellent reputation to have a healthy body. Fish meat is extremely rich in omega 3-fatty acids, and they are also packed with other healthy nutrition that helps to reduce inflammation from the body. Fishes including, salmon, snapper, cod, tuna, bass, and halibut, are all very rich in healthy fats. Salmon is the only fish that has

EPA and DHA are the omega-three fatty acids that produce anti-inflammatory molecules.

4) Allium Vegetables

Allium vegetables, also known as Anti-inflammatory vegetables. The word "Allium" is a Latin word for "Garlic." Humans have been using garlic for several years now. Despite being so old, these vegetables still do miracles in saving us from chronic inflammatory diseases. The allium vegetables include Garlic, Onion, Chives, Shallots, Scallions, and leeks. These vegetables are packed with many healthy nutrients. The onions A is a molecule that significantly helps in reducing inflammation from the body. The molecule is present in Onions.

5) Gluten-Free Grains

Quinoa has become the most popular gluten-free grains. It's a rich source of fiber and helps with inflammatory diseases. The second product is Brown Rice, that has significant importance in controlling the sugar levels of the body. As proven from the research, replacing white rice with brown rice have drastically added many health benefits.

6) Root Vegetables

The root vegetables are not only delicious, but they are also packed with healthy nutrition. The root vegetables such as sweet potatoes, parsnips, rutabaga, and beets are loaded with immune-boosting vitamins.

Carrots are one good source of vitamin A, whereas sweet potatoes consist of compounds that are helpful for digestion. Along with digestion, these vegetables also help with the vision, encourages the immune system, and keeps skin glowing.

7) Berries

As mentioned earlier, fruits are known for their anti-inflammatory properties. So, the berries are also one good source of anti-oxidants

8) Dark leafy greens

Dark leafy greens are rich in anti-oxidants. They are packed with Vitamin A, Vitamin C, Vitamin E, and Vitamin K. Dark leafy greens are fully packed with omega 3 fatty acids that aid digestion and also very good for the nervous system.

9) Nuts & seeds

Nuts like walnuts and seeds like chia seeds are the best for inflammation in the body. These two are packed with proteins and fibers and are also very rich in Omega 3 fatty acids.

10) Ginger

Ginger has "anti-inflammatory" properties. It has a compound named "gingerols" that inhibits anti-inflammatory molecules. It is also used to treat several medical conditions like digestion problems, arthritis, headaches, cold, and many others.

HEAL YOUR GUT

To cut a long story short, these inflammatory diseases can be reduced to a drastic level just by adopting a healthy diet. The anti-inflammatory diet is the one that keeps your body away from inflammation.

The basic guideline to follow is:

1. Eat enough fruits and vegetables

2. Eat food with higher sources of fat

3. Always strike a balance between Omega 3 & Omega 6 fatty acids

4. Eat food that supports your gut

5. Stay away from artificial sugars and processed foods

6. Drink enough water to keep yourself hydrated

7. Last but not least, get enough sleep of 6-8 hours.

Now we move on to the Diet-Plans

The Vegan Diet Plan

The vegan Diet Plan consists of fruits, vegetables, nuts, seeds, and oil. Please be careful and try not to use any animal products in this diet.

1) Eat Enough Fruits & Vegetables

Eat enough fruits and vegetables to get all the anti-inflammatory nutrients. Once you adopt such a routine, you will see a positive change in your health.

2) Eat plant-based protein

Plant-based protein is vital to have an anti-inflammatory nutrient. Some vegans are known as "Carbotarians." They eat pasta, brown rice, bread, and baked items. The plant-based protein is essential to eat as it helps in repairing and healing damaging tissue.

3) Omega 3 fatty Acid Intake

Eat foods that have plenty of Omega 3 fatty acids. The omega 3 fatty acids help with the digestion process. Eat nuts, seeds, along with fresh vegetables.

4) Avoid processed foods

The people on vegan diets often tend to develop a craving for something tasty. As a result, they opt for processed vegan food, with the texture of animal foods like vegan chicken, tuna, sausages etc. Our advice for such vegans is not to opt for this option. The processed food contains artificial flavors, preservatives, and that has nothing healthy in it. Also, the non-dairy products, including yogurt, cheese, are all thickened with artificial stabilizers named carrageenan. The carrageenan is a chemical compound that is responsible for inflammation in the body.

5) Eat Gluten-free grains

Eat food that is gluten-free and stay away from gluten products. Eat brown rice instead of white rice, eat healthy grains, and don't go for something that will cause inflammation in the body.

As we have seen, eating healthy is not a matter of strict limitations; staying too thin or resisting food that you love the most. It's more about feeling good, having more energy, improving your health, and improving your mood.

Healthy eating should not be too difficult to acquire. If you feel astounded by all the conflicting advice on nutrition and diet, you are not the only one. You will find out that for every expert who tells you that a particular food is right for you, you will find another that says precisely the opposite. The truth is that, although it has been shown that certain specific foods or nutrients have a beneficial effect on mood, the most important thing is your general diet. The foundation of a healthy diet should be to replace processed foods with real foods whenever possible. Eating food as close as possible to the way nature has prepared it can make a significant difference in the way you think, look, and feel.

Proteins give you the energy to get up and leave and continue while assisting the mood and thought process. Too much protein can be life-threatening to people with kidney disease, but the latest research suggests that many of us need more high-quality protein, especially as we get older. It does not mean that you need to eat more animal products: a variety of vegetable sources of protein every day can provide your body with all the essential proteins it needs.

To prepare for success, try to keep it simple. Healthy eating does not have to be difficult. Instead of worrying too much about calorie counting, for example, think about your diet in terms of food color, variety, and freshness of food. The focus should be on avoiding packaged and processed foods and opt for fresher ingredients whenever possible.

Chapter 03: 14-Day Meal Plan & Protocols to follow

Inflammation is the normal process triggered by the person's body in response to any illness, toxins, and as a result of chronic disease. It's a short term process, but if not dealt properly, it can result in long term inflammation. It can be so ruthless that it can cause or trigger severe health conditions. The chapter presents a 14-Day meal plan that aims to reduce inflammation.

The essentials of the anti-inflammatory diets are based on :

- Limiting extra sugar

- Limited refined products

- Avoiding cooking procedures that cause inflammation

To reduce inflammation, a person should eat such foods that provide anti-oxidants as these are the one prime factor to reduce inflammation from the body.

The anti-inflammatory diet is all about consuming foods that help to decrease inflammation in the body.

When we limit the foods that tend to increase inflammation, we began to fight inflammatory health conditions. The anti-inflammatory diet stresses lots of vibrant fruits and vegetables, high-fiber beans and whole grains, healthy fats (like the ones found in salmon, nut and olive oil), and antioxidant-rich herbs, spices, and tea.

We must limit processed foods that have unhealthy trans fats, refined carbohydrates like "white flour" and "white sugar," which also contain much sodium in them.

We are offering a 1,200-calorie meal plan, in which we pull everything together to provide you the week full of delicious, healthy meals and snacks. Our diet plan will allow you to have a successful and healthy life.

The inflammation can be triggered by several other factors apart from food, like reduced activity levels, stress, and insufficient sleep. Adopting a healthy lifestyle and added healthy habits into your daily life can also help prevent inflammation.

To have the maximum anti-inflammatory benefits, couple this healthy meal plan with your daily physical activity that aims for around 2 1/2 hours of reasonable activity per week, and opt for activities that helps to reduce inflammation as yoga, meditation or whatever you find relaxing, and try to have enough sleep every night (at least 6-7 hours every night. Even if you're working to decrease inflammation vigorously or are simply looking for a healthy eating plan, the 7-day anti-inflammatory meal plan can help you in achieving your health goals.

Anti-Inflammatory Diet (Day 01):

Eat foods that are rich in omega-3 fatty acids, such as salmon and albacore tuna, and sardines have been shown to drop inflammation levels. The diet plan aims to include at least two "3-ounce servings" of fish having high levels of omega-3 fatty acids and consume every week.

Breakfast, "287 calories."

- One serving of Blueberry-Banana Overnight Oats

- One cup of green tea

Afternoon Snacks, "31 calories."

- 1/2 cup of blackberries

Lunch Time, "325 calories."

- One serving of Green Salad with Edamame & Beets

Evening Snack, "117 calories."

- Two Tbsps. of Turmeric-Ginger Tahini Dip

- one medium carrot

Dinner "442 calories."

- One serving of Walnut-Rosemary Crusted Salmon

- One serving Roasted Squash & Apples with Dried Cherries & Pepitas

Total Calories and Nutrition: 1,202 calories, 57 g protein, 131 g carbohydrate, 30 g fiber, 54 g fat, 1,520 mg sodium.

Anti-Inflammatory Diet (Day 02):

Day 02 includes eating foods that contain Vitamin C, which is an antioxidant and has anti-inflammatory effects. Vitamin C helps in decreasing damaging free radical cells that might activate inflammation. It has been proven that people having diets rich in vitamin C have reduced levels of the inflammatory marker C-reactive protein as well as the minor risk of inflammatory disease, including gout and heart diseases. The diet includes Raspberry-Kefir Power Smoothie that provides 45 percent of the recommended percentage of Vitamin C consumption

Breakfast, "249 calories."

- One serving of Raspberry-Kefir Power Smoothie

Afternoon Snack, "28 calories."

- 1/3 cup of blueberries

Lunch "381 calories."

- One serving of Vegan Superfood Buddha Bowl

Evening Snack, "156 calories."

- 1 ounce of dark chocolate

Dinner "393 calories."

- one serving of Indian-Spiced Cauliflower & Chickpea Salad

- 5 ounces of unsalted canned albacore tuna, in water (drained)

Total Calories & Nutrition: 1,215 calories, 70 g protein, 143 g carbohydrate, 35 g fiber, 47 g fat, 1,054 mg sodium

Anti-Inflammatory Diet (Day 03):

The third day includes eating Anthocyanin, which is a strong antioxidant compound found in dark-colored fruits and vegetables such as red, purple, and blue. The antioxidant is also found in red wine. As per the research, anthocyanin plays a significant role in reducing inflammation markers that can reduce health risks related to cancer and heart diseases. Eat frozen berries to provide an anti-inflammatory aid to your morning smoothies or oatmeal. By having berries, you can get the maximum benefits even apart from the season.

Breakfast, "263 calories."

- 1 cup of low-fat plain Greek yogurt

- 1 1/2 of Tbsp. chopped walnuts

- 1/4 of cup blueberries

- 1 cup of green tea

Add yogurt with nuts and blueberries to enhance the taste

Afternoon Snack, "42 calories."

- 2/3 cup of raspberries

Lunch "381 calories."

- one serving of Vegan Superfood Buddha Bowl

Evening Snack, "117 calories."

- 2 Tbsp. of Turmeric-Ginger Tahini Dip
- one medium carrot

Dinner "409 calories."

- one serving of Superfood Chopped Salad with Salmon & Creamy Garlic Dressing

Total Calories and Nutrition: 1,212 calories 77 g protein, 97 g carbohydrate, 28 g fiber, 63 g fat, 813 mg sodium

Anti-Inflammatory Diet (Day-04):

Day 04 consists of eating dark chocolate and cocoa. Chocolate tends to cut inflammation markers, and it's really helpful in reducing heart diseases. Cocoa has flavonol quercetin, which is a powerful antioxidant, and it helps in protecting our cells, and that's the reason dark chocolate is an essential element in the anti-inflammatory diet plan. Include one 1-ounce square a day of the darkest chocolate and enjoy the maximum health benefits.

Breakfast, "222 calories."

- One serving of Cocoa-Chia Pudding with Raspberries

Afternoon Snack, "109 calories."

- 1/2 cup of low-fat plain Greek yogurt
- 1/4 cup of blueberries

Lunch "381 calories."

- One serving of Vegan Superfood Buddha Bowl

Evening Snack, "9 calories."

- 1/2 cup of sliced cucumber

- Pinch of salt

- Pinch of pepper

Dinner "472 calories."

- one serving of Stuffed Sweet Potato with Hummus Dressing

Total calories and Nutrition: 1,191 calories, 56 g protein, 168 g carbohydrate, 49 g fiber, 39 g fat, 1,100 mg sodium.

Anti-Inflammatory Diet (Day-05):

Probiotics have been found to have tremendous health benefits and are proven to be an excellent source to reduce inflammation. These are found in yogurt, kefir, kombucha, and kimchi and greatly helps in maintaining a healthy gut. As per the research, healthy gut mends our immune systems; it helps in sustaining a healthy weight and significantly reduces inflammation. Besides, make sure to add prebiotics that are indigestible plant fibers found in garlic, onions, and whole grains. It provides ignition to good bacteria and improves overall gut health.

Breakfast, "249 calories."

- one serving of Raspberry-Kefir Power Smoothie

Afternoon Snack, "2 calories."

- one cup of green tea

Lunch "381 calories."

- one serving of Vegan Superfood Buddha Bowl

Evening Snack, "58 calories."

- 1 Tbsp. of Turmeric-Ginger Tahini Dip

- 3/4 cup of sliced cucumber

Dinner "414 calories."

- one serving of Korean Steak, Kimchi & Cauliflower Rice Bowl

Total Calories and Nutrition: 1,224 calories, 57 g protein, 112 g carbohydrate, 28 g fiber, 53 g fat, 1,067 mg sodium

Anti-Inflammatory Diet (Day 06)

It has been observed that around 21 percent of adults from all over the U.S have some sort of arthritis. It's an inflammatory disease that hits the joints. The disease is generally treated with prescribed medicines along with the anti-inflammatory diet. Such diets that are rich in magnesium have been known to reduce inflammation and greatly helps in maintaining joint cartilage. Many of the people living in the U.S don't get a sufficient amount of magnesium, and as a result, they tend to suffer more from the disease. Make sure to include legumes, nuts, and green leafy vegetables in your diet to gain the maximum health benefits.

Breakfast, "249 calories."

- One serving of Raspberry-Kefir Power Smoothie

Afternoon Snack, "157 calories."

- 06 walnuts

Lunch "325 calories."

- one serving of Green Salad with Edamame & Beets

Evening Snack, "78 calories."

- 1/2 ounce of dark chocolate

Dinner "401 calories."

- one serving of Hummus-Crusted Chicken
- one serving of Blistered Broccoli with Garlic and Chiles

Tip: Cook an extra spare chicken for lunch tomorrow. You'll be needing 2 cups of chopped cooked chicken.

Total Calories and Nutrition: 1,209 calories, 73 g protein, 94 g carbohydrate, 28 g fiber, 63 g fat, 1,245 mg sodium

Anti-Inflammatory Diet (Day-07):

As per the research, a diet with rich fiber in it has reduced levels of the glycemic index. It is a way of measuring how does food impacts our blood sugar levels. Fiber digests slowly; as a result, it keeps us filled and maintains blood sugar levels. Also, foods that have a lower glycemic index greatly help to reduce C-reactive protein levels, which is known as inflammation indicator. With the help of this plan, a person can easily have around 28g of fiber and can enjoy the health benefits.

Breakfast, "292 calories."

- One serving of Cocoa-Chia Pudding with Raspberries

- One Turmeric Latte

Afternoon Snack, "42 calories."

- 1/2 cup of blueberries

Lunch "350 calories."

- One serving of Avocado Egg Salad Sandwiches

Evening Snack, "116 calories."

- 15 almonds (unsalted)

Dinner "448 calories."

- One serving of One-Pot Garlicky Shrimp & Spinach

- One cup of cooked quinoa

Total Calories and Nutrition: 1,209 calories, 62 g protein, 128 g carbohydrate, 32 g fiber, 55 g fat, 1,362 mg sodium

Second-Week Meal Plan

Calorie calculation is a tough job. We don't always have the option of measuring calories as far as our diet is concerned. So the second-week meal plan offers a diet plan, which you can have in your routine without actually measuring the calories for it. It's a diet plan you can trust to reduce inflammation from the body.

We all know that food plays a major part in controlling inflammation from the body. So, we have gathered some of the anti-inflammatory recipes. All the recipes mentioned in this diet plan will help to reduce the inflammation from the body.

Anti-Inflammatory Diet Plan (Day-01)

Breakfast: "Cherry Coconut Porridge"

Porridges are known as traditional breakfast. Some people add cherries (dried or fresh) in their porridge which is an excellent idea. Cherries contain anthocyanin, which is a powerful antioxidant, and people have been using anthocyanin to reduce inflammation for quite sometime

Recipe:

- 1.5 cups of Oats
- 4 tablespoons of Chia Seeds
- 3-4 cups of Coconut Milk
- 3-4 tablespoons of Cacao (raw)
- A pinch of Stevia
- Coconuts
- Free cherries or frozen
- Shavings of Dark Chocolate
- Maple Syrup

Preparation: Mix oats with chia seeds, milk (coconut), cacao, and stevia in a pan. Boil it over medium heat and then boil on lower heat till oats are cooked.

Once it is cooked, pour this into the bowl and add coconut shavings, cherries, dark chocolate shavings, and maple syrup on top to make it taste good.

Lunch: "Thai Pumpkin Soup"

Pumpkins are known as the rich source of beta-cryptoxanthin. It is a strong antioxidant and worked best when absorbed with fat, and makes butter and oil important in this recipe to make it more than just a flavor. Pumpkin Skins are eatable, and it makes the preparation very stress-free. Enjoy the soup with a healthy green salad and gain the maximum benefits from it.

Recipe:

- 2 tablespoons of red curry paste

- 4 cups of broth (chicken or vegetable broth)

- 2 and a half ounces "Pumpkin-Pree Cans."

- 1 ¾ cups of milk (coconut)

- Chili pepper sliced (one)

- Cilantro for decoration, if required

Preparation:

Step 01: Cook the curry paste for about 1 minute or until the paste becomes fragrant in a large pan on medium heat. Now add broth and pumpkin and gently stir.

Step 02: Cook for about 3 minutes or until soup starts to bubble. Add the coconut milk and cook until hot, about 3 minutes.

Step 03: Now serve into bowls and relish with a sprinkle of the coconut milk and red chilis slice. In the last, garnish it with cilantro if you want it. Enjoy the healthy soup to reduce inflammation from the body

Dinner: "Curried Potatoes with Poached Eggs"

Eggs can't be used only for breakfast. Poached Eggs when served with potatoes and green salad becomes a very healthy dinner. The reason why eggs are recommended is that they are rich in Omega-3-Fatty acids, and these acids are known as the ones with anti-inflammatory properties. We can use this healthy dinner to reduce the inflammation from the body.

Recipe:

- 02 Russet potatoes

- 1" inch fresh ginger

- 2 garlic cloves

- 1 tablespoon of Olive Oil

- 2 tablespoons of hot or mild curry powder

- 15-ounce tomato sauce can

- 4 eggs (large)

- Half bunch fresh cilantro, if needed

Preparation:

Step 01: Rinse the potatoes thoroughly, then cut them into 3/4-inch cubes. Now place the potatoes in a pot and cover it with water. Cover up the pot with a lid and boil on high heat. Keep boiling potatoes for 5-6 minutes, or until they're tendered.

Step 02: When the potatoes are boiling, prepare the sauce. Peel ginger with a vegetable peeler or scrape the skin off with spoon sides. Use cheese grater with small holes to grate one inch of ginger or less if you like subtle flavor of ginger. And grind the garlic

Step 03: Now add garlic, olive oil, and ginger into a big pot. Cook the ginger and garlic on medium-low heat for about 1-2 minutes, or just until it is soft and fragrant. Now mix curry powder to it and cook for about 01 minutes or more to toast the spices.

Step 04: Now mix the tomato sauce into it and stir gently. Heat up to medium and heat the sauce. Add salt if it is needed. Now insert the cooked and tender potatoes to the pot and stir to cover in the sauce. Add a few tablespoons of water if the mixture is dry or pasty.

Step 05: Make four small dips in the potato mixture and add an egg into each. Cover the pan and let it boil. After boiling the eggs in the sauce for about 6-10 minutes, or until they are well-cooked, sprinkle it with chopped fresh cilantro.

Anti-Inflammatory Diet-Plan (Day 02)

Breakfast: "Raspberry Smoothie"

If you want a quick and healthy breakfast, don't worry. We have a "Raspberry Smoothie" that not only provides you with the anti-inflammatory benefits, but it also tastes good. You can also have the option of making this smoothie and store in the fridge. Just drink it before you step out of the door.

Recipe:

- peeled avocado or pitted if you want
- 3/4 cup of orange juice
- 3/4 cup of raspberry juice
- 1/2 cup of raspberries

Preparation:

Now add all the ingredients mentioned above mix them well and enjoy your healthy smoothie. It's a drink full of anti-oxidants, and it will certainly reduce inflammation from the body up to a significant level.

Lunch: "Mediterranean Tuna Salad"

Tuna is very famous for its benefits. It's a rich source of Omega-3 Fatty acids. You can have it with mixed greens or grain bread. The recipe that we are going to share is rich in sodium, so you can always have the option of scaling it down by decreasing the number of capers and olives.

Recipe:

- 2 "5-ounces" cans tuna in drained water

- 1/4 cup of mayonnaise

- 1/4 cup of chopped kalamata or mixed olives

- 2 Tablespoons of chopped red onion

- 2 Tablespoons of minced fire-roasted red peppers

- 2 Tablespoons of chopped fresh basil

- 1 Tablespoon of capers

- 1 Tablespoon of fresh lemon juice

- salt and pepper as needed

- 2 big vine-ripened tomatoes

Preparation:

Mix all the ingredients excluding tomatoes in a large pot then stir gently to mix. Cut tomatoes into sixths, without cutting them all, then gently open. Now empty Mediterranean Tuna Salad mixture from the center. Now serve the Mediterranean Tuna Salad to enjoy the maximum health benefits.

Dinner: "Slow Cooker Turkey Chili"

In colder evenings, nothing keeps you warm but chili. When mixed with Turkey, it becomes the best combination to eat at dinner. It not only helps you keep warm but also helps to reduce the inflammation from the body.

Recipe:

- 1 tablespoon of olive oil

- 1 pound of 99% lean ground turkey

- 1 medium onion chopped

- 1 red pepper diced

- 1 yellow pepper diced

- 2 "15-ounce" cans tomato sauce

- 2 "15-ounce" cans petite chopped tomatoes

- 2 "15-ounce" cans black beans,

- 2 "15-ounce" cans red kidney beans, washed and drained

- 1 "16-ounce" jar deli-sliced tamed jalapeno peppers, drained

- 1 cup of frozen corn

- 2 tablespoons of chili powder

- 1 tablespoon of cumin

- Salt and black as per the requirement

Suggested toppings: green onions cheese, avocado, sour cream/Greek yogurt

Preparation:

Heat the oil in a pot on medium heat. Add turkey in the pot, and cook until it turns brown. Now pour turkey in the slow cooker.

Add the tomato sauce, onion, chopped tomatoes, beans, jalapeños, peppers, corn, chili powder, and cumin. Stir and sprinkle with salt and pepper.

Now cover it and let it cook on High for about 4 hours or on low heat for 6 hours. Serve it with toppings, if wished.

Anti-Inflammatory Diet Plan (Day-03)

Breakfast: "Gingerbread Oatmeal"

As we all know that Omega 3-Fatty Acids are the main ingredients when it comes to reducing inflammation of arthritis, and many other joints problems. We need to look for ways from where we get the maximum Omega 3-fatty acids. Oatmeal can suffice half of the requirement of omega 3-fatty acids, without salmon in it.

Recipe:

- 4 cups of water

- 1 cup of steel-cut oats

- 1 and 1/2 tablespoon of ground cinnamon

- 1/4 tablespoon of ground coriander

- 1/4 tablespoon of ground cloves

- 1/4 tablespoon of ground ginger

- 1/4 tablespoon of crushed allspice

- 1/8 tablespoon of ground nutmeg

- 1/4 tablespoon of ground cardamom

- maple syrup to enhance the taste

Preparation: Prepare the oats to package directions and also add the spices when you mix the oats in the water.

When you are finished cooking, mix maple syrup to enhance the taste.

Lunch: "Kale Caesar Salad with Grilled Chicken"

Roasted chicken is very easy to find in the supermarket. It not only tastes delicious but also saves time and allows you to make quick meals. This time when you go to buy, pick two, one for dinner and the other one for lunch. It is also known to have anti-inflammatory properties.

Recipe:

- 8 ounces of grilled chicken, finely sliced

- 6 cups of curly kale, cut into small sized pieces

- 1 cup of cherry tomatoes, sliced

- 3/4 cup of shredded Parmesan cheese

- Half coddled egg "cooked about 1 minute."

- 01 garlic clove, crushed

- Half teaspoon of Dijon mustard

- 1 teaspoon of honey

- 1/8 cup of fresh lemon juice

- 1/8 cup of olive oil

- freshly ground black pepper and Kosher salt

- 2 Lavash of flatbreads or two large tortillas

Preparation:

In a pot, mix the half of a coddled egg, crushed garlic, mustard, honey, lemon juice, and olive oil. Beat until you have made a dressing. Add salt and pepper to augment the taste.

Now add the kale, chicken and cherry tomatoes and mix to cover it with the dressing and ¼ cup of the shredded parmesan.

Spread the two lavash flatbreads. Equally, distribute the salad with the two wraps and powder each with ¼ cup of parmesan.

Roll the wraps, cut it into half and eat instantly

Dinner: "Baked Tilapia with Pecan Rosemary topping."

Tilapia is an excellent source of Selenium. It's a mineral proved to help patients with Arthritis. The good thing about this meal is, it can be easily and quickly cooked, and it's enough for the whole family to enjoy. It can also be prepared if you want to eat a fancier meal. Don't worry if you don't want to eat tilapia; you can replace it with trout or cod.

Recipe:

- 1/3 cup of sliced raw pecans

- 1/3 cup of whole-wheat panko bread crumbs

- 2 teaspoons of minced fresh rosemary

- Half teaspoon of coconut palm sugar (also brown sugar if you want)

- 1/8 teaspoon of salt

- 1 pinch of cayenne pepper

- One and a half teaspoon of olive oil

- One egg white

- 4 "4-ounces" tilapia fillets

Preparation:

Before preparing this meal, preheat the oven to a temperature of 350 degrees F.

Take a small baking dish, mix pecans, breadcrumbs, rosemary, coconut palm sugar, salt, and cayenne pepper together. Now add olive oil and mix to cover the pecan mixture.

Start Baking till the pecan mixture turns light golden brown, it takes about 7 to 8 minutes.

Increase the temperature of the oven to 400 degrees F. Cover a large glass baking dish with cooking spray.

In a narrow dish, beat the egg white. Take one tilapia fillet at a time, dip the fish in egg white and then the pecan mixture, and lightly cover each side. Put the fillets in the prepared baking dish.

Now put the remaining pecan mixture on top of the tilapia fillets.

Start Baking until the tilapia is well-cooked, it takes about 10 minutes to cook properly.

Anti-Inflammatory Diet-Plan (Day-04)

Breakfast: "Rhubarb, apple, and ginger muffins."

By far, we get the idea that ginger is a great source to reduce inflammation in the body, and it also helps to comfort arthritis pain. With mixed with apple and Rhubarb, it becomes a healthy breakfast to eat.

Recipe:

- 1/2 cup of ground almonds

- 1/4 cup of raw sugar (unrefined)

- 2 tablespoons of lightly sliced crystallized ginger

- 1 tablespoon of ground linseed meal

- 1/2 cup of buckwheat flour

- 1/4 cup of fine brown rice flour

- 2 tablespoons of organic cornflour

- 2 teaspoons of gluten-free baking powder

- 1/2 teaspoon of crushed cinnamon

- 1/2 teaspoon of crushed ginger

- a decent pinch fine sea salt

- 1 cup finely of sliced rhubarb

- 1 small apple, cored and finely sliced

- 1/3 cup with 1 tablespoon of rice or almond milk

- 1/4 cup of olive oil

- 1 big egg

- 1 teaspoon of vanilla extract

Preparation:

Now preheat the oven to a temperature 180C/350C. Oil 1/3 cup capacity muffin tins with paper cases.

Put almonds, sugar (raw), ginger, and linseed meal to a medium-sized pot. Add over flours, baking powder, and spices, then beat to combine them. Stir in rhubarb and apple to cover in the flour mixture. Take another smaller bowl and whisk oil, egg milk, and vanilla before pouring this into dry mixture and stir. Equally, divide the batter between paper cases (spread with a few slices of rhubarb if needed) and bake for about 20-25 minutes, until risen, golden around the edges and when a skewer is put into the center, it comes out clean. Now remove it from the oven and wait for about 5 minutes and allow it to cool. Eat warm or at room temperature.

Anti-Inflammatory Diet Plan (Day-05)
Breakfast: "Buckwheat and Ginger Granola"

This meal is certainly packed with some of the best anti-inflammatory ingredients. When topped with Almond milk, this granola even tastes better. The breakfast is healthy, anti-inflammatory, and energizing as well.

Recipe:

- 1 cup of Buckwheat

- 2 cups of rolled oats (Gluten-free)

- 1 cup of sunflower seeds

- 1 cup of pumpkin seeds

- One and a half cup of dates

- 06 tablespoons of coconut oil

- 04 tablespoons of cacao powder (raw)

- 1 inch of ginger root

Preparation:

1. Pre-heating the oven to 180C

2. Put the oats, buckwheat, and seeds into a large bowl and stir gently

3. Now add dates, coconut oil, and apple pieces into a pan and boil them for five minutes, until the dates become soft

4. Once the dates are cooked, peel the ginger and grate it; once it's grated, mix it with dates.

5. Once the dates are fluffy, put them into a blender with the raw cacao powder and blend until the mix is smooth (including the coconut oil, ginger and apple puree)

6. After this, pour the mixture over the buckwheat, oat and seed mix and blend well to make sure everything is coated.

7. Oil one large baking tray with coconut oil and spread

the granola out over them.

8. Put the baking trays in the oven and bake for around 45 minutes. Stir after every 15 minutes

9. Once it's nice and crispy, make sure not burning, take the granola out of the oven, and let it cool and place it in an airtight container to store.

Lunch:" Roasted Red Pepper & Sweet Potato Soup"

The soup contains anti-oxidants and will greatly help inflammatory symptoms

Recipe:

- 2 tablespoons of olive oil

- 2 onions, minced

- 1 jar (12-ounces) roasted red peppers (chopped)

- 1 can (4-ounces) green chiles (chopped)

- 2 teaspoons ground cumin

- 1 teaspoon of salt

- 1 teaspoon of ground coriander

- 3 to 4 cups peeled, diced sweet potatoes

- 4 cups of vegetable broth

- 2 tablespoons of fresh cilantro (crushed)

- 1 tablespoon of lemon juice

- 4 ounces of cream cheese, diced

Preparation:

Take large soup pot, heat the olive oil on medium-high heat. Add onions and cook until its soft. Now add red peppers, cumin, salt, green chilies, and coriander. Cook them for 1 to 2 minutes.

Now mix the reserved juice from the roasted red peppers, sweet potatoes, and vegetable broth. Boil them, reduce the heat and cover. Cook for about 10 to 15 minutes stir in the cilantro and lemon juice. Allow it to cool.

Place half of the soup into a mixer along with the cream cheese. Blend until it's smooth, add salt if needed, and your dish is ready.

Dinner: "Lemon Herb Salmon & Zucchini"

Salmon is widely known for its anti-inflammatory properties. The dinner we are going to prepare has salmon and undoubtedly the best taste.

Recipe:

- 4 zucchinis, sliced

- 2 tablespoons of olive oil

- Kosher salt and ground black pepper, to enhance the taste

- 2 tablespoons of brown sugar

- 2 tablespoons of lemon juice (fresh)

- 1 tablespoon of Dijon mustard

- 2 garlic cloves, minced

- Half teaspoon of dried dill

- Half teaspoon of dried oregano

- 1/4 teaspoon of dried thyme

- 1/4 teaspoon of dried rosemary

- 4 (5-ounce) salmon fillets

- 2 tablespoons of parsley leaves (freshly chopped)

Preparation:

Preheat the oven up to 400 degrees. Slightly oil a baking sheet

Take a small bowl and beat brown sugar, lemon juice, Dijon, garlic, dill, oregano, thyme, and rosemary together & add salt and pepper to taste.

Put zucchini in a single layer. Sprinkle with olive oil and add salt and pepper to taste. Now add salmon in a single layer and brush every filet with a mixture (herb)

Put this into the oven and cook about 16 to 18 minutes.

Anti-inflammatory Diet Plan (Day-06)

Breakfast: "Baby Spinach & Mushroom Frittata"

This meal has mushroom and spinach that are packed with nutrition

Recipe:

- 06 eggs

- 1/4 cup of milk (60ml)

- 1 cup grated cheddar cheese ((250 ml)

- 1 onion, sliced

- 4 ounces of white button mushrooms, sliced

- 3 tablespoons of butter

- 2 cups of baby spinach

- Salt and pepper to taste

Preparation:

Preheat the oven to 180 °C or (350 °F). Butter a 20-cm four-sided baking dish.

Take a large bowl, mix eggs and milk with a beater. Now add cheese. Also, put salt and pepper as per your requirement

In a large non-stick pot, brown onion and mushrooms in butter on medium heat. Sprinkle salt and pepper. Now add spinach and cook for about 1 minute, continuously stirring.

Add mushroom mixture into the egg mixture. Stir fine and put it into a baking dish. Bake the frittata around 25 minutes or until slightly browned. Slice the frittata into four squares and remove them from a dish.

Lunch: "Smoked Salmon Potato Tartine"

Recipe:

- 1 large potato

- 2 tablespoons of butter

- kosher salt

- black pepper

- 4 ounces of soft goat cheese

- One and a half tablespoons of finely chopped chives

- Half garlic clove, thinly sliced

- Lemon for taste

- finely sliced smoked salmon

- 2 tablespoons of drained capers

- 2 tablespoons of finely sliced red onion

- 1/2 hardboiled egg

- Thinly chopped chives (for garnish)

Preparation:

Mix goat cheese, lemon, and garlic in a small bowl. Sprinkle with salt and pepper to taste. Slightly stir in fresh chives.

Sprinkle the chopped red onion and hard-boiled egg with salt.

Grate the potato using large holes of a grater. Sprinkle generously with salt and pepper.

Start heating the butter in a small non-stick pot over medium to high heat. Once it's hot, add grated potato

Suppress the mixture with the back of a spoon to make it compact, cook slowly for about 8-10 minutes each side

Allow it to cool until hardly lukewarm or room temperature.

When potato cake has cooled, add goat cheese mixture on the top. Layer the smoked salmon on this and drizzle with the red onion, hardboiled egg, and capers.

Dinner: "Sweet Potato Black Bean Burger"

Recipe:

- 2 cups of mashed sweet potato

- 1 cup of cooked salted black beans

- One and a half cup of brown rice (cooked)

- Half cup walnut

- Half cup of thinly chopped green onion

- 2 and a 1/2 teaspoon of ground cumin

- 1 teaspoon of paprika (smoked)

- 1/4 teaspoon of salt and pepper for taste

Preparation:

Preheat the oven to 204 C. Cut sweet potatoes in half. Brush with olive oil and put it face down on a baking sheet. Bake sweet potatoes until tender for about 30 minutes and decrease the heat

Cook rice or quinoa while potatoes are baking

Put black beans in a mixing bowl and mash half of them for texture. Now add the sweet potato and lightly mash, then 1 cup rice, green onion, nut meal, and spices. Mix everything to combine.

Lightly oil a baking sheet and mark a 1/4 cup with plastic wrap.

Fill the marked measuring cup with sweet potato mixture.

Bake burgers for about 30-45 minutes, with carefully flipping after 20 minutes to make sure each side is cooked.

Anti-Inflammatory Diet Plan (Day-07)

Breakfast: "Gluten-Free Crepes"

Recipe:

- 02 eggs

- 1 teaspoon of vanilla (gluten-free)

- Half cup of nut milk

- Half cup of water

- 1/4 teaspoon of salt

- 1 or 2 tablespoons of agave nectar

- 1 cup of flour (Gluten-free)

- 2 tablespoons of coconut oil (melted)

- 1 tablespoon of coconut oil

Preparation:

Put 02 tablespoons of coconut oil into a small pan, and

heat over low heat to melt

Take a mixing bowl and beat the eggs, vanilla, nut milk, water, salt, and agave nectar until they are combined well.

Gently add in the flour and beat to combine

Now remove the oil from heat, and put into the batter in a steady stream while mixing slowly

Pour the batter onto the cook, using approximately 1/3 cup for each crepe.

The moment you poured the batter, tilt the pan in a circular motion so that the batter coats evenly

Cook the crepe for 2 minutes and serve.

Lunch: "Red Lentil and Squash Curry Stew"

Recipe:

- 01 tablespoon of Extra virgin olive oil (EVOO)

- 01 sweet onion, sliced

- 03 garlic cloves chopped

- 1 tablespoon of curry powder

- 1 carton of broth

- 1 cup of red lentils

- 3 cups of cooked butternut mash

- 1 cup of greens

- grated ginger, for taste (optional)

Preparation:

Take a large pot, add EVOO and sliced onion, and chopped garlic. Cook for about 5 minutes on low to medium heat.

Mix in curry powder and cook another couple of minutes. Add broth and lentils and heat till it boils

Mix cooked butternut squash and greens. Cook over medium heat for about 5-8 minutes. Sprinkle with salt, pepper, and add freshly grated ginger to enhance the taste.

Dinner: "Turkey & Quinoa Stuffed Bell Peppers"

- 3 medium-sized yellow peppers

- 1.25 pounds extra lean ground turkey

- 1 cup of diced mushrooms

- 1/4 cup of diced sweet onion

- 1 cup of sliced fresh spinach

- 2 teaspoons of crushed garlic

- 1 (1 8 ounces) can of tomato sauce

- 1 cup of chicken broth

- 1 cup of dry quinoa

Preparation:

Take a small saucepan, start with quinoa and cook as per the instructions on the pack (usually about 15 minutes).

While the quinoa cooks, pan-fry the vegetables with a little butter or olive oil.

After about 5 minutes or so, add ground turkey and garlic into the vegetables. Prepare over medium heat. Once the turkey is mostly cooked, though, put tomato sauce and about half of the chicken broth in it. Prepare until the turkey is entirely cooked.

Preheat the oven to 400.

As the turkey mixture boils, prepare your bell peppers. Wash the peppers, slice them in half, and get rid of the stem & seeds. Spray baking pan with cooking spray and place the sliced bell peppers in the pan

Once the quinoa is prepared, put it into the pan with the turkey & vegetables. Mix. Then, fill each bell pepper with the mixture. Make sure they are nicely filled! And your dish is ready to serve.

Chapter 04: Tips & Tricks to continue the Healing Journey

The subject of inflammation is the most commonly discussed. Every other person you meet is dealing with some sort of chronic inflammatory disease, including joint pains and arthritis. However, to fight against such chronic diseases is not that challenging, then it appears. All you need to do is to opt. for a healthy lifestyle.

The hype created by inflammatory diseases has positive reasons. Adopting an anti-inflammatory diet will not only reduce chronic inflammation, but it will also help you to stay fit and healthy in the long run. As per the research, it can also decrease the risk of heart attack, dementia, and diabetes.

The good thing is that you don't have to wait for years to see healthy results. The small tips and tricks that we are going to mention in the book will help you reduce inflammation overnight. All you need to do is to adopt these tricks or habits to remain healthy and fit, and you can easily continue the healing journey effortlessly.

1) Eat green salad daily.

Always buy a pack or two of leafy greens to mix for your meals. The leafy greens are very beneficial; having a cup full of leafy greens as baby spinach, arugula, kale, or lettuce daily is one of the most useful diet habits you can adopt. The leafy greens provide an anti-inflammatory benefit, as they contain antioxidants and bioactive compounds that have the potential to reduce inflammation and also inhibits free radicals from generating new inflammation in the body.

2) Avoid artificial flavors.

Avoid the vending machine and artificially sweetened drinks, and go for a fiber-rich food with a little protein in it as apple slice, peanut butter, raw vegetables, and hummus, or eat a handful of almonds and cheese cubes. The reason why it is important is that having a balanced food without artificial sugars and refined carbs are essential to keep your blood sugar under normal parameters, which in the long run will help you to deal with cravings, hunger, and bowel irritability. It will keep you fit and healthy and is also beneficial for the people around you. Limiting peaks and drops in blood sugar helps you to inhibit inflammation in the body that can lead to obesity, diabetes (Type 02), and many other heart diseases.

3) Sleep on Time.

Turn off the television, close all the social media applications, and move to bed a little earlier than you sleep. It might appear a bit indulgent, but to have at least 7 to 8 hours of uninterrupted sleep is what's required and considered sufficient for grownups, and we should all have a sufficient sleep to stay healthy. Not getting enough sleep (6 hours or less) daily activates inflammation, even if you are healthy. The research advocates increased risk for metabolic issues that could lead to obesity, diabetes (Type 2), and many other heart diseases, dementia, and Alzheimer's as well.

4) Don't forget to walk daily.

Have you ever missed your workout? Don't worry, and take a speedy walk around the block! Although regular exercise is perfect for dealing and preventing almost every health issue, some days, we don't have enough time for a full-scale workout. On the other hand, research advocates that having just 20-25 minutes of muscle movement can reduce inflammatory blood markers. So, tie up your shoes and start running.

5) Add Flavors in Food.

There is always a way to make the food more delicious and spicy, even if you are following a diet. Find out ways to mix a little garlic or spice when you're preparing the dinner tonight. Aromatic and strong spices look like they have the potential to augment inflammation, but research advises the opposite, most of them are proven healthy. There is enough evidence to recommend adding garlic, or herbs and spices, including turmeric, rosemary, cinnamon, cumin, ginger, and fenugreek, which reduces inflammation in the body that could ultimately lead to heart diseases, other brain degenerative conditions, cancer, and respirational issues.

6) Stay Away from Liquor.

If you want to have an evening cocktail or glass full of wine, think of withholding for a couple of days. It doesn't have to be lasting, but avoiding alcohol for as many days as you can help to reduce inflammation from the body. Besides, cutting out liquor helps the body to stay calm, and also it reduces existing inflammation. According to some researchers, having reasonable alcohol consumption has some health benefits; the only problem is that it is not easy to maintain the line between advantageous and anti-inflammatory to destructive and inflammatory.

7) Swap your coffee with green tea.

If you are habitual of drinking 1 to 3 cups of coffee or other caffeinated juices daily, think of substituting one of those with a cup of green tea instead. Green tea leaves are filled with polyphenol compounds that can significantly help in decreasing free radical destruction to stop additional inflammation. The research advocates that regular consumption of green tea can help decrease your risk of Alzheimer's disease, cancer, and joint problems.

8) Be very kind to your gut.

There's lots of hysteria about probiotics, but do you support those good microbes already existing in you? Shelter the existing good bacteria by cutting out artificial sugars, trans fats, and always focus on picking primarily whole and slightly processed foods. It is also worth having food that is rich in probiotics—like yogurt, sauerkraut, kombucha, miso, or kimchi—daily. Encouraging the gut's microbe obstruction is one of the foundations to reduce inflammation from the body in the long-run.

9) Try Fasting occasionally

Although it's not for everyone, many of the researchers claim to find benefits when it comes to having intermittent fasting (IF), mostly because of the anti-inflammatory impacts, the eating pattern develops. There are many ways to fasting, but the easiest means to start is with a 12-hour fast. It means if you have taken your dinner at 7 p.m., then you only have water or anything you want to eat till 7 a.m. the next morning. As per the researches, frequently having IF also reduce heart disease risk and increases insulin sensitivity, brain health, and inflammatory bowel disease.

10)Stay Away from dairy and gluten products

Dairy and gluten are not commonly inflammatory in healthy people (unless you are allergic, intolerant, or have celiac disease), but these products can be annoying when there's already inflammation in the body. Many people find it helpful to eliminate dairy, gluten, or both these products for a couple of weeks while having a diet rich in anti-inflammatory foods and low in inflammatory ones. The reason behind it is that it gives the body some time to remain calm. After this, you can gradually begin to add dairy or gluten-containing foods to check if they cause any sort of irritation.

11) Take some time to Relax.

It doesn't matter whether you have a healthy diet or not, if stress levels are constantly high, low-grade inflammation is going to stay. Even though if increased stress levels are not much of everyday concern, learning how to manage and deal when it does happen is vital to prevent new inflammation in the body. Find healthy means or methods to escape that pressure and anxiety, for example, practicing yoga daily, meditation is also very good, or you can also take short walks as it offers rapid relief mentally and anti-inflammatory effects physiologically.

12)Be very selective with ingredients.

Flavors, dyes, artificial preservatives, and many other elements frequently added to meals, all have a greater possibility to activate or augment inflammation — specifically if you have a weak gut barrier. So, it is always better to have a look at the ingredient side of products placed in your store and fridge. Are the ingredients mentioned what you could have possibly used if you were making the meal from a recipe at home? If yes, then it is probably a negligibly processed product and an upright choice. If it is not, then opt for

another product or substitute when you go shopping
next time.

Chapter 05: Delicious & Healing Recipes

The reason to have an anti-inflammatory diet is not to lose weight, so it shouldn't be considered as a "diet" in the traditional use of that term. As per the research, an anti-inflammatory diet pattern consists of meals and recipes that can naturally reduce inflammatory markers in the body. In simple words, the anti-inflammatory diet is purely the one that will not make your body suffer an immune response.

1. "Baked Sweet Potatoes (with Tahini Sauce)"

- 4 medium-sized sweet potatoes
- 1 "15-ounce can" of chickpeas (washed)
- Half Tablespoon of olive oil
- Half tsp of each cumin, coriander, cinnamon, and paprika
- 1 pinch of sea salt or lemon juice (Not necessary)
- 1/4 cup of hummus (or tahini)
- Medium lemon (half)
- 3/4 or 1 tablespoon of dried dill
- 3 garlic cloves, minced

Preparation:

Preheating the oven to 400 degrees F (204 C)

Wash and scrub potatoes and cut in half lengthwise

Sprinkle rinsed and drained chickpeas with olive oil and spices

Scrub the sweet potatoes with a bit of olive oil and place face down on the same baking sheet

While sweet potatoes and chickpeas are frying, prepare the sauce by mixing all ingredients to a bowl and beating to combine, only adding water to almond milk to thin. Taste and adjust flavors as needed.

Once sweet potatoes are soft, and the chickpeas are golden brown remove from oven after 25 minutes.

For serving, flip the potatoes flesh part up and smash down the insides a little bit. Then top with chickpeas, sauce, and parsley-tomato garnish. Enjoy your food.

2. "Artichoke Ricotta Flatbread."

- Half pound homemade pizza dough

- olive oil

- on and a half cup of fresh whole milk ricotta cheese

- 2 tablespoons of fresh basil chopped

- 1 tablespoon of honey

- 8 ounces of marinated artichokes (drained)

- 6 ounces of fresh mortadella

- 3 cups of fresh arugula

- Half cup of fresh parmesan cheese

- 1 tablespoon of fresh chives

Lemon Vinaigrette

- 1/3 cup of olive oil

- juice and pulp of 1 lemon

- 2 teaspoons of apple cider vinegar

Preparation:

Preheat the oven to 450 degrees F.

On a lightly floured surface, roll the dough out until it is very slim. Move the dough to the prepared baking sheet and sprinkle with olive oil and also drizzle with salt and pepper. Place in the oven and bake for 8-10 minutes

For now, mix the ricotta, basil, honey, and a pinch of both salt and pepper. Take the bread from the oven and top with the ricotta. Toss on the artichokes and then drizzle with crushed red pepper flakes, if wished. Top with fresh arugula and parmesan. A moment before serving sprinkle lemon vinaigrette, chives and ENJOY

3. "Lemon chicken with asparagus."

- 1 pound of boneless chicken breasts
- 1/4 cup of flour

- 1/2 teaspoon of salt, pepper to enhance the taste

- 2 tablespoons of butter

- 1 teaspoon of lemon pepper flavor

- 1 to 2 cups minced asparagus

- 2 lemons, cut in halves

- 2 tablespoons of honey and 2 tablespoons butter (if interested)

- parsley for topping (as per choice)

Preparation

Cover the chicken breasts with a plastic wrap and strike until every piece is about a 3/4 of an inch.

Add the flour, salt, and pepper in a dish and smoothly mix each chicken breast in the dish for covering. Boil down the butter in a large pot on medium-high heat; Now add the chicken and cook it around 3 to 5 minutes (each side), until it changes color, drizzling each side with the lemon pepper straight in the pan. When the chicken has finally turned golden brown and cooked well, transfer it to a plate.

Now insert the minced asparagus to the pan. Cook for a few minutes until it's crispy. Take out from the pan and set aside. Put the lemon slices flat at the bottom of the pan and sauté for a few minutes on every side without stirring so that it can be caramelized and pick up the toasted bits left in the pan from the chicken and butter. Take out the lemons from the pan and set aside.

Coat all the ingredients back into the pan – asparagus, chicken, and lemon slices on the top and enjoy the dish

4. "Walnut sage pesto pasta with roasted delicata squash."

- 2 medium-sized delicata squash, scrubbed and rinsed well

- 2 tablespoons of extra virgin olive oil

- Sea salt

- black pepper

- 1 or 2 packed cup of flat-leaf parsley leaves

- 3/4 cup toasted walnut halves

- 2 to 3 garlic cloves (medium-sized)

- 6-7 large and fresh sage leaves

- Half cup roasted of walnut oil

- fresh sage leaves, to Fry

- 1/4 cup extra of virgin olive oil

- 1 pound of dried whole wheat penne

- Half cup finely grated "Parmigiano Reggiano" cheese,

Preparation

Preheat the oven to 425 degrees Fahrenheit.

Neat the ends of the delicata squash and cut them in half lengthwise. Use a spoon to scoop out the seeds and remove them. Slice each half into 1/2-inch of half-moon portions and put on the sheet pan. Sprinkle with olive oil, salt, and pepper, and lay them out evenly on the sheet pan. Cook at 425 degrees for about 20 to 25 minutes, Flip the squash halfway through, until its cooked

While the squash is cooking, make the walnut-sage pesto. Mix the parsley leaves, walnuts, garlic cloves, and fresh sage leaves in the bowl Mix the roasted walnut oil and continue to mix until it's smooth. Flavor to taste with salt and pepper, and move to a bowl.

Then fry the sage leaves, in bunches, in the oil until its crisp. Move with a slotted spoon to the bowl and flavored slightly with salt.

By now, the squash is done roasting, Insert the dried whole wheat pasta to the boiling water and cook well. Spare roughly a cup of the pasta cooking water. Now transfer the pasta back to the same pan, Sprinkle lightly with olive oil, and mix. Now insert the walnut-sage pesto and grated Parmigiano-Reggiano cheese and mix till the pasta is evenly covered in the sauce. Add some of the reserved pasta water if required

Serve the pasta topped with roasted Delicata squash pieces, and have fun.

5. "Shawarma Salad (Chicken)"

- 1 "5-ounce can" of chickpeas
- 1 Tablespoon of olive oil
- 1 teaspoon of cumin
- A half heaping teaspoon of smoked paprika
- A half heaping teaspoon of turmeric
- Half slight teaspoon sea salt for taste
- Half teaspoon of ground cinnamon
- 1/4 teaspoon of ground ginger
- 1 pinch of black pepper, ground coriander, and cardamom
- 5 ounces spring mix lettuce (organic)
- 10 cherry tomatoes (sliced)
- 1/4 cup of red onion (finely sliced)
- 3/4 cup of fresh parsley
- 20 pita chips

Preparation

Heat the oven to 400 degrees F (204 C) and place a stand in the middle of the oven.

Insert cleaned and dried chickpeas to a mixing dish.

Now add olive oil and all flavors and mix to combine them.

Section a chickpea and adjust flavors as per the requirement. Now position in a single layer on a bare baking sheet and bake for about 20 to 22 minutes, or until it changes color.

Meanwhile, it's cooking, make salad ingredients and place them to a bowl

For the dressing, mix hummus, garlic, dill, and lemon juice to a small mixing dish and beat to combine. Then add lukewarm water till it becomes pourable and serve.

6. "Sheet Pan Shrimp Fajitas"

- 1 and a half pounds of shrimp
- 1 yellow bell pepper thinly sliced
- 1 red bell pepper thinly sliced
- 1 orange bell pepper thinly sliced
- 1 small red onion thinly sliced
- 1 and a half tbsp. of extra virgin olive oil
- kosher salt to taste
- freshly ground pepper
- 2 teaspoon chili powder
- 1/2 teaspoon garlic powder
- 1/2 teaspoon onion powder
- 1/2 teaspoon ground cumin
- 1/2 teaspoon smoked paprika
- Lime and fresh cilantro for garnish
- tortillas (warmed)

Preparation

Preheat oven to 450 degrees

Take a large bowl and combine, shrimp, olive oil, salt,

onion, bell pepper and pepper and spices for the taste

Now mix them to combine.

Sprinkle the baking sheet with cooking spray. (nonstick)

Place shrimps, bell peppers, and onions on a baking sheet.

Saute at 450 degrees for around 8 minutes. Now turn oven to broil and allow it to cook for extra 2 minutes or until shrimp is cooked well.

Now add juice from a fresh lime over fajita blend and top with fresh cilantro and serve.

7. "Tomato Garlic Basil Chicken"

- 1 pound of boneless chicken breasts
- 2 tablespoons of olive oil
- Half yellow onion, chopped
- 3 minced garlic cloves
- 15 ounces can of Italian sliced tomatoes
- one handful of fresh basil,
- 1/4 teaspoon of minced red pepper flakes
- 4 medium-sized zucchini, courgette, covered into spaghetti-like noodles

Preparation

Wrap the chicken with plastic and strike each piece to make it even, for about one inch. Once finished, drizzle each side with a little salt and pepper.

Insert 1 tablespoon olive oil into a large pot, until its warm. Now add the chicken in it and pan fry every side until it changes the color.

When the chicken is cooked well and changed color, take it from the pot

Use the same pot again and add remaining olive oil and cook the onion until it becomes soft around 5 minutes. Now insert the garlic and cook for one minute more. Put the tomatoes and basil into the skillet and flavor with the salt, pepper, and red pepper flakes.

Sauté for about 10 more minutes until the sauce becomes thin. Make sure to stir in between.

Put chicken back to the pot along with the noodles to marinate in the sauce a few minutes and then serve.

8. "Spaghetti Squash with Asparagus, Ricotta, Lemon, and Thyme"

- 1 "1/2 pounds" of small spaghetti squash
- 1 tablespoon of olive oil
- 2 crushed cloves garlic,
- 1 pound of asparagus
- 3/4 cup of ricotta cheese
- 3 tablespoons of freshly squeezed lemon juice
- 1 teaspoon of slightly grated lemon pulp
- 1 teaspoon of fresh thyme leaves
- Half teaspoon of kosher salt
- 1/4 teaspoon of black pepper
- 3 tablespoons of toasted pine nuts

Preparation

Preheat the oven to 375°F. Place the frame in the middle of the oven

Slice the squash in half lengthwise and remove the seeds. Coat the slices with 1/2 tablespoon of the oil. Put the slices down on one half of a baking sheet. Cook for about 35 minutes. In the meantime, neat the woody sides of the asparagus

Take out the baking sheet with the squash, mix the asparagus to the other side, and mix with the remaining half tablespoon of oil. Put a garlic clove under each squash half. Get back to the baking sheet to the oven and cook until the asparagus is cooked well, and squash is a tender fork; it will take around 10 minutes. In the meanwhile, put the zest, thyme, salt, ricotta, lemon juice, and pepper in a large dish and stir gently combine.

Remove the baking sheet from the oven and cautiously remove the garlic cloves from under the squash. Add to the ricotta and mix fine. Add the asparagus to the bowl, and your dish is ready to serve.

9. "Butternut Squash & Kale Farro Risotto"

- 1 cup of Farro
- 2 cups of Boiling Water

- 5 cups of Chicken Stock low-sodium

- 2 and a half cups of butternut Squash chopped into small chunks

- 1 bunch Kale sliced

- 3 Tablespoons of Olive Oil

- 2 Shallots, chopped

- 2 crushed garlic cloves

- Half cup of dry White Wine

- 1 Tablespoon of Unsalted Butter

- 1/2 cup of Parmesan

- 1/4 cup of pecorino Romano

- 1 Tablespoon of Lemon Juice

- Salt and Pepper (to taste)

Preparation

Add the two cups of boiling water over the farro in a container and allow it soak for at a few hours

Dry the farro well and position it into a high-speed blender

Cook the chicken stock in a skillet on high until it starts boiling

Once it is boiled, turn the heat down to low, cover, and let it cook

Take a large frying pan, heat the two tablespoons of olive oil on medium heat

Cook the shallots until it changes color

Add the garlic in it and cook until it changes color to light brown

Add in the crushed farro, make sure that all the farro is covered in the oil

Add half cup of white wine and mix until the wine has mostly cooked off

Turn the heat down to medium heat and add in about 1/4 cup of broth at the same time, repeatedly stir the farro risotto till the liquid has completely absorbed

Continue adding 1/4 cup of broth at the same time and stir gently until the broth has been used completely

When the broth has been mixed into the risotto, in about 30 minutes, take it away from the heat and combine with the Parmesan, Pecorino Romano, butter, lemon juice, salt, and pepper, butternut squash, and kale and your food is ready to be served.

Final Words

Thank you again for purchasing this book!

We really hope this book is able to help you.

The next step is for you to **join our email newsletter** to receive updates on any upcoming new book releases or promotions. You can sign-up for free and as a bonus, you will also receive our "*7 Fitness Mistakes You Don't Know You're Making*" book! This bonus book breaks down many of the most common fitness mistakes and will demystify many of the complexities and science of getting into shape. Having all this fitness knowledge and science organized into an actionable step-by-step book will help you get started in the right direction in your fitness journey! To join our free email newsletter and grab your free book, please visit the link and signup: **www.cffingopublishing.com/gift**

Finally, if you enjoyed this book, then we would like to ask you for a favor, would you be kind enough to leave a review for this book? It would be greatly appreciated! Thank you and good luck in your journey!

About the Co-Authors

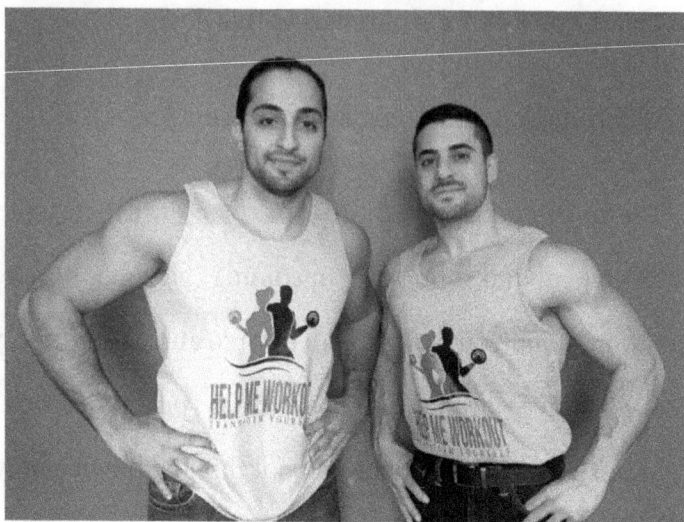

Our name is Alex & George Kaplo; we're both certified personal trainers from Montreal, Canada. Will start off by saying we are not the biggest guys you will ever meet and this has never really been our goal. In fact, we started working out to overcome our biggest insecurity when we were younger, which was our self-confidence. You may be going through some challenges right now, or you may simply want to get fit, and we can certainly relate.

For us personally, we always kind were interested in the health & fitness world and wanted to gain some muscle due to the numerous bullying in our teenage years. We figured we can do something about how our body looks like. This was the beginning of our transformation journey. We had no idea where to start, but we both just got started. We felt worried and afraid at times that other people would make fun of us for doing the exercises the wrong way. We always wished we had a friend to guide us and who could just show us the ropes.

After a lot of work, studying and countless trial and errors. Some people began to notice how we were both getting more fit and how we were starting to form a keen interest in the topic. This led many friends and new faces to come to us and ask us for fitness advice. At first, it seemed odd when people asked us to help them get in shape. But what kept us going is when they started to see changes in their own body and told us it's the first time that they saw real results! From there, more people kept coming to us, and it made both of us realize after so much reading and studying in this field that it did help us but it also allowed us to help others. To date, we have coached and trained numerous clients who have achieved some pretty amazing results.

Today, both of us own & operate this publishing business, where we bring passionate and expert authors to write about health and fitness topics. We also run an online fitness business and we would love to connect with you by inviting you to visit the website on the following page and signing up to our e-mail newsletter (you will even get a free book).

Last but not least, if you are in the position we were once in and you want some guidance, don't hesitate and ask... will be there to help you out!

Your coaches,

Alex & George Kaplo

Download another book for Free

We want to thank you for purchasing this book and offer you another book (just as long and valuable as this book), "Health & Fitness Mistakes You Don't Know You're Making", completely free.

Visit the link below to signup and receive it:

www.effingopublishing.com/gift

In this book, we will break down the most common health & fitness mistakes, you are probably committing right now, and will reveal how you can easily get in the best shape of your life!

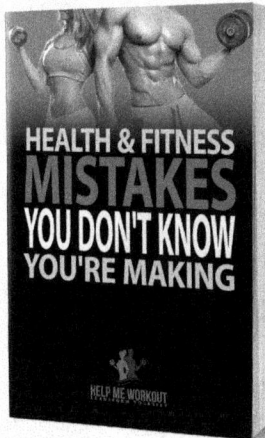

In addition to this valuable gift, you will also have an opportunity to get our new books for free, enter giveaways, and receive other valuable emails from us. Again, visit the link to sign up:

www.effingopublishing.com/gift

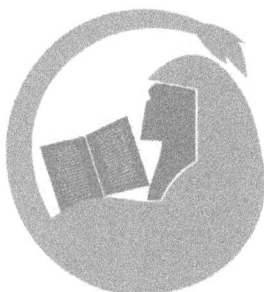

EFFINGO
Publishing

For more great books visit:

EffingoPublishing.com